INSULIN RESISTANCE RECIPES FOR BEGINNERS

Transform Your Diet, Control Blood Sugar, Boost Energy, And Embrace Wellness With Flavorful Dishes Meal Plans And Expert Tips

DR. JACE ZAYDEN

Table of Contents

DISCLAIMER

The information provided in the book is intended for general informational purposes only. The content of this book should not be considered a substitute for professional medical advice, diagnosis, or treatment.

Readers are advised to consult with a qualified healthcare professional for medical advice tailored to their individual circumstances.

The author has made every effort to ensure that the information in this book is accurate and up-to-date at the time of publication. However, medical knowledge is constantly evolving, and new research may emerge that could impact the information presented. The author disclaims any responsibility for any adverse effects or consequences resulting from the use of the information provided in this book.

References or mentions of individuals, products, websites, organizations, or other names within this book are for informational purposes only and do not constitute an endorsement. The author has no affiliations with, and makes no endorsements of, any third-party entities mentioned. Readers are encouraged to conduct their own research and exercise their judgment when considering any external resources or recommendations.

The author and the publisher shall have neither liability nor responsibility to any person or entity with respect to any loss, damage, or injury caused or alleged to be caused directly or indirectly by the information contained in this book. Any reliance on the information within this book is at the reader's own risk.

By reading this book, the reader acknowledges and agrees to the terms of this disclaimer. If the reader does not agree with these terms, they should not use the information provided in this book.

ABOUT THIS BOOK

This book "Insulin Resistance Recipes" is an exceptionally valuable resource for those who are afflicted with insulin resistance. It offers an exhaustive understanding of the condition and practical solutions in the form of a compilation of meticulously crafted recipes. The introductory section provides an overview of the foundational principles underlying insulin resistance, thereby establishing a solid foundation for the subsequent discussion. This scientific book "Understanding Insulin and Its Role" clarifies the critical function of insulin within the body.

Significant attention is devoted to the "Importance of a Balanced Diet," which underscores the critical function that nutrition fulfills in the management of insulin sensitivity. This book comprehensively covers a range of meal categories, commencing with "Insulin-Friendly Breakfast Recipes" and advancing to "Wholesome Lunch Options" and "Nutrient-Rich Snack Ideas." A holistic approach to sustaining a balanced diet is exemplified by the incorporation of "Dinner Recipes to Support Insulin Sensitivity" and "Desserts and Treats for Insulin-Resistant Individuals" as well.

This book offers recommendations on beverage selections and the importance of "Meal Planning" to optimize the management of insulin resistance, in addition to recipes. The inclusion of practical recommendations regarding "Incorporating Exercise into Your Routine" and "Lifestyle Changes for Managing Insulin Resistance" broadens the scope beyond dietary modifications, providing a holistic approach to overall health.

"Grocery Shopping Guide" and "Sample Meal Plans" facilitate the incorporation of insulin-friendly options into meal preparation, whereas "Cooking Techniques for Insulin Resistance" guarantees that the meal preparation is by health objectives. "Frequently Asked Questions" (FAQs) and "Common Myths and Facts about Insulin Resistance" debunk prevalent misunderstandings, respectively, and provide answers to inquiries.

"Insulin Resistance Recipes" serves as more than a mere cookbook; rather, it functions as a comprehensive manual that enables readers to exercise discernment when it comes to the management of insulin resistance. Through the integration of scientific knowledge and pragmatic resolutions, this book transforms into an indispensable resource for individuals grappling with the intricacies of insulin resistance, facilitating a path toward enhanced physical and mental health.

CHAPTER ONE

An Overview Of Insulin Resistance

Insulin resistance is a metabolic disorder characterized by an impaired cellular response to the hormone insulin, which is secreted by the pancreas. Insulin is an indispensable hormone in the regulation of blood sugar (glucose) levels through its facilitation of glucose cell absorption. Glucose cannot access cells efficiently when they develop resistance to the effects of insulin; this results in elevated blood sugar levels.

Eventually, the pancreas may produce more insulin to mitigate for its diminished efficacy due to this resistance. This increased insulin secretion may, with time, contribute to a range of health complications, such as obesity, type 2 diabetes, and cardiovascular disease. Insulin resistance is frequently associated with genetic factors, obesity, and a sedentary lifestyle.

It is critical to comprehend the mechanisms underlying insulin resistance to effectively manage and prevent the associated health complications. Dietary and other lifestyle modifications are crucial in the treatment of insulin resistance.

Comprehension Of Insulin And Its Function

Insulin functions as a key that grants access to cells for glucose, which supplies energy. Glucose accumulates in the bloodstream when cells resist this key, resulting in elevated blood sugar levels. This condition may contribute to the development of type 2 diabetes if left untreated; it can cause fatigue and increased appetite.

Diet is a significant determinant of insulin resistance. Insulin resistance can be worsened by diets that are high in refined carbohydrates and sugars, which induce swift increases in blood glucose levels. Cells gradually lose their sensitivity to insulin signals.

Besides dietary components, genetics, sedentary occupations, and obesity are additional determinants of insulin resistance.

Consistent engagement in physical activity enhances insulin sensitivity, thereby increasing cellular responsiveness to its signals. Ensuring a healthy weight is of paramount importance in the management of insulin resistance, given that elevated insulin resistance is correlated with surplus fat, especially in the abdominal region.

The Value Of A Well-Balanced Diet

A well-balanced diet is fundamental to the management of insulin resistance. The process entails the selection of nutrient-dense foods that supply vital vitamins, minerals, and fiber while preventing significant fluctuations in blood glucose levels. It is crucial to prioritize whole, unprocessed foods over refined and high-sugar alternatives.

A varied selection of fruits, vegetables, lean proteins, and whole cereals incorporated into one's diet promotes overall health and aids in blood sugar regulation. The sluggish absorption of glucose by foods high in fiber prevents rapid surges and declines.

Additionally, nutritious lipids, including those present in avocados and almonds, contribute to the regulation of blood sugar.

When considering insulin resistance, the importance of meal planning increases significantly. By incorporating well-balanced meals and refreshments into one's daily caloric intake, it is possible to effectively regulate blood sugar levels consistently. The implementation of portion control and mindful dining is crucial to fostering weight management and deterring excessive consumption.

Recipes For Insulin-Friendly Breakfast

Breakfast is frequently regarded as the most vital meal of the day, and individuals who are managing insulin resistance can capitalize on this by consuming a well-balanced meal. Protein, nutritious lipids, and complex carbohydrates, when consumed together, can help regulate blood sugar levels and provide sustained energy.

1. Yogurt Parfait In Greece:

• Greek yogurt, assorted berries, pistachios, and a drizzle of honey are the components.

• To prepare, arrange Greek yogurt, berries, and hazelnuts in a glass; drizzle a small amount of honey on top.

2. Omelette Of Vegetables:

• Eggs, spinach, tomatoes, bell peppers, and feta cheese are the ingredients.

• Whisk the eggs before adding them to the sautéed vegetables in a saucepan. Feta cheese enhances the flavor of an omelet.

3. Chia Seed Confection:

• Sliced strawberries, chia seeds, almond milk, and vanilla extract are the ingredients.

• Incorporate chia seeds, almond milk, and vanilla into the mixture. Refrigerate overnight, and in the morning, garnish with strawberries.

Nutritious Lunch Alternatives For Individuals With Insulin Resistance

Including a diverse array of nutrients in one's lunch provides a favorable occasion to promote holistic well-being and effectively regulate insulin resistance. Three nutritious lunch alternatives are as follows:

1. Quinoa and Grilled Chicken Salad:

• Quinoa, grilled chicken breast, cucumber, feta cheese, and a lemon vinaigrette are the components.

• To prepare the dish, preheat the quinoa, combine it with the diced vegetables, and garnish with grilled chicken, feta, lemon juice, and olive oil vinaigrette.

2. Wrap of salmon and avocado:

• A whole-grain wrap, seared salmon, avocado slices, lettuce, and Greek yogurt sauce are the ingredients.

• Assemble the components within the wrap, garnish with Greek yogurt sauce, and savor a meal that is rich in essential nutrients.

3. Bowl of Vegetarian Buddha:

Brown rice, roasted sweet potatoes, chickpeas, sautéed kale, and tahini vinaigrette are the components.

• Procedure: assemble the components in a bowl, garnish with tahini vinaigrette, and savor a delectable and vibrant supper.

In summary, the effective management of insulin resistance necessitates a comprehensive strategy encompassing consistent physical activity, weight maintenance, and judicious dietary selections. Individuals can acquire knowledge regarding the function of insulin, the significance of maintaining a balanced diet, and the integration of insulin-friendly recipes into their daily meals, thereby engaging in proactive measures that promote overall health and wellness.

Recipes For Insulin Resistance: Nurturing Your Body For Equilibrium

Insulin resistance is a pathological state characterized by decreased cellular responsiveness to the regulatory effects of insulin, ultimately resulting in hyperglycemia. Managing insulin resistance frequently necessitates dietary and other lifestyle modifications. It is essential to increase insulin sensitivity and promote overall health by developing recipes for snacks, dinners, desserts, and beverages that are abundant in nutrients and resistant to insulin.

CHAPTER TWO

Ideas For Nutrient-Dense Snacks: Intelligently Fueling Your Body

Snacking is a crucial component in the management of insulin resistance. Snacks that are rich in nutrients can aid in blood sugar regulation and prevent energy declines.

For sustained energy, choose munchies that consist of a combination of protein, healthy fats, and complex carbohydrates.

1. Greek Yogurt Parfait: Begin with a sprinkling of fruit and unsweetened, pure Greek yogurt; garnish with a pinch of nuts or seeds. Antioxidants, protein, and probiotics are abundant in this refreshment.

2. Vegetable Sticks with Hummus: Accompany a portion of hummus with sliced, vibrant vegetables such as bell peppers, carrots, and cucumbers. Hummus provides a substantial amount of protein and healthful lipids, both of which aid in satiety.

3. Crackers Made with Whole Grain and Avocado: For a scrumptious nibble, spread pureed avocado on whole grain crackers. The monounsaturated lipids found in avocados have the potential to enhance insulin sensitivity.

4. Hard-boiled eggs serve as a practical and nutrient-dense refreshment option. In addition to stabilizing blood sugar levels, they can prolong satiety between meals.

5. Chia Seed Pudding: Soak chia seeds in almond milk for the duration of the night. Add berries or almonds as a garnish for a delectable and fiber-rich refreshment.

Dinner Dishes That Promote Insulin Sensitivity: A Harmonious Combination Of Flavors And Nutrition

Developing well-balanced dinner recipes is crucial for individuals who are undergoing insulin resistance management. Adopt a diet rich in lean proteins, whole cereals, and vegetables to stabilize blood sugar levels and promote optimal nutrition.

1. Quinoa and Roasted Vegetables with Grilled Salmon is an excellent source of omega-3 fatty acids, which possess anti-inflammatory qualities. Complement it with an assortment of roasted vegetables and quinoa to create a nutrient-dense entrée.

2. Stir-Fried Turkey and Vegetables: In a stir-fry, combine a variety of vibrant vegetables with lean turkey. Herbs, seasonings, and minimal oil are sufficient to create a delectable, insulin-friendly meal.

3. For a balanced dinner, prepare chicken breasts that have been baked and garnished with roasted sweet potatoes and steamed broccoli. For the chicken breasts, sprinkle them with seasonings.

4. Concoct a substantial vegetarian chickpea curry that combines an abundance of vegetables with a delectable blend of seasonings. For added fiber, serve it over brown rice or quinoa.

5. Zucchini Noodles with Pesto and Grilled Shrimp: For a low-carb, insulin-friendly dinner

option, substitute traditional pasta with zucchini noodles, garnish with homemade pesto, and add grilled shrimp.

Desserts And Treats For Insulin-Resistant Individuals: A Healthy Way To Satisfy Your Sweet Tooth

It is crucial to discover alternatives to traditional desserts that do not cause a rise in blood sugar levels when managing insulin resistance. Select delicacies that incorporate nutrient-dense ingredients and utilize natural sweeteners.

1. Berry and Yogurt Parfait: For a delectable dessert that is also rich in probiotics and antioxidants, arrange an assortment of berries on a parfait made with Greek yogurt and a touch of honey.

2. Clusters of Dark Chocolate and Nuts: To create gratifying clusters, combine dark chocolate with nuts such as almonds or walnuts. Antioxidants present in dark chocolate potentially improve insulin sensitivity.

3. Apples Baked with Cinnamon: Scatter cinnamon over apples that have been cored and baked until tender. This straightforward confection is fiber-rich and naturally delicious.

4. Chia Seed Chocolate Pudding: Employ chia seeds, cocoa powder, and a natural sweetener to make a chocolate pudding. This dessert is rich in healthful lipids and fiber.

5. Coconut and Almond Energy bits: To make energy bits, combine shredded coconut, almond butter, and a dash of honey. These portable delights are composed of a blend of protein and healthful fats.

Adequate Hydration For Individuals With Insulin Sensitivity

Beverage selection is an essential factor in the management of insulin resistance. Choosing low-sugar, hydrating alternatives is crucial for one's overall health.

Include the following:

1. Hydrate with pure water or, for added flavor, a dash of lemon juice. A well-hydrated body is beneficial for overall health and may assist in the management of insulin sensitivity.

2. Herbal Teas: Indulge in the flavor and warmth of herbal teas such as ginger, peppermint, or chamomile, which do not contain added carbohydrates.

3. Green tea is rich in compounds and antioxidants that have the potential to enhance insulin sensitivity. Provide it as an option for a refreshing beverage.

Avoid the following:

1. Avoid sugar-sweetened beverages such as energy drinks, fruit juices, and sodas, as they have the potential to cause abrupt increases in blood glucose levels.

2. Coffee beverages that are laden with sugar and high-calorie syrups should be avoided. Choose

black or naturally sweetened alternatives to coffee sweeteners.

3. In contrast to the potential health advantages associated with moderate alcohol consumption, excessive ingestion can have detrimental effects on blood sugar levels. If possible, consume alcohol in moderation.

Insulin Resistance Meal Planning Advice: Constructing A Balanced Plate

Effective meal planning is essential for managing insulin resistance. Here are some suggestions for preparing insulin-friendly and well-balanced meals:

1. Placing Emphasis on Whole Foods: To ensure a diverse array of nutrients, opt for unprocessed, whole foods that are whole, including lean proteins, whole cereals, fruits, vegetables, and healthy lipids.

2. Portion Control: To prevent excess, pay close attention to portion sizes. By balancing

carbohydrates with lipids and proteins, blood sugar levels can be better regulated.

3. Promote Satiety and Blood Sugar Stabilization: Incorporate dietary fiber into your diet by consuming vegetables, fruits, legumes, and whole grains, all of which are rich in fiber.

4. Opt for Healthier Fat Sources: Give precedence to consuming healthy fats, including avocados, almonds, seeds, and olive oil, as they have the potential to elevate insulin sensitivity.

5. Consume balanced, fewer meals and nibbles spaced out throughout the day to mitigate significant fluctuations in blood sugar levels.

6. Maintain Consistency: To aid in the regulation of insulin production and the maintenance of stable blood sugar levels, establish a consistent meal schedule.

In summary, the process of formulating recipes for managing insulin resistance necessitates deliberate selections that promote holistic health and welfare. Through the incorporation of nutrient-dense munchies, well-balanced dinners, gratifying desserts, hydrating beverages, and strategic meal planning, individuals can foster a healthier lifestyle and effectively manage insulin sensitivity. It is advisable to consistently seek personalized guidance from a registered dietitian or healthcare professional regarding specific dietary requirements.

CHAPTER THREE

A Gastronomic Method For Health Management

Insulin resistance occurs when the cells of the body develop a diminished sensitivity to the regulatory hormone insulin, which is responsible for controlling blood sugar. It is a precursor to type 2 diabetes and has been associated with a range of health complications. The management of insulin resistance necessitates a comprehensive strategy, with dietary modification that promotes stable blood sugar levels constituting a critical component. In this article, we shall explore recipes for managing insulin resistance that prioritize whole, nutrient-dense foods, to assist you in preparing palatable and health-conscious meals.

When formulating recipes for individuals with insulin resistance, prioritize ingredients that have a low glycemic index (GI). The gradual release of glucose into the circulation by foods with a low glycemic index prevents rapid increases in blood sugar. Blend nutritious lipids, lean proteins, and vegetables abundant in fiber to produce well-balanced meals. The following is an illustrative recipe to commence your preparations:

Salmon grilled in the presence of roasted vegetables

The following are the ingredients:

Salmon fillets—four

(2) teaspoons of extra virgin olive oil

(1) teaspoon juice of citrus

• 1 teaspoon garlic, minced

• Pepper and salt to flavor

• Four cups of assorted vegetables (zucchini, cherry tomatoes, bell peppers, etc.)

• 1 tablespoon vinegar balsamic

• Herbs young for garnish

Means of instruction:

1. Preheat the oven and grill to medium-high temperatures.

2. Combine olive oil, lemon juice, minced garlic, salt, and pepper in a small basin. Apply this mixture to the salmon fillets using a brush.

3. Cook the salmon for four to five minutes per side, or until thoroughly cooked.

4. Combine the vegetables and toss them with balsamic vinegar, pepper, and salt. Preheat them until tender in the oven.

5. Present the seared salmon atop the roasted vegetables with fresh herbs as a garnish.

Integration Of Physical Activity Into One's Regimen: An Essential Elements In The Management Of Insulin Resistance

Physical activity is an efficacious strategy for regulating insulin resistance, given its capacity to enhance insulin sensitivity and foster general well-being.

It is not difficult to incorporate regular physical activity into one's routine; modest adjustments to one's lifestyle can yield substantial results. The following suggestions will assist you in incorporating exercise into your daily life:

1. Select Pleasurable Activities: Whether it be gardening, cycling, walking, or dancing, identify pursuits that you sincerely take pleasure in. This enhances the probability that you will maintain a long-term commitment to them.

2. Commence Gradually: Commence exercising gradually if you are new to it or have been inactive for an extended period. Start with brief sessions and increase the duration and intensity progressively as your fitness level improves.

3. Integrate Cardiovascular and Strength Training: An all-encompassing exercise regimen incorporates resistance training and cardiovascular activities.

Weight-bearing cardiovascular exercises such as brisk walking and jogging are beneficial to the heart, whereas strength training increases muscle mass and metabolism.

4. Establish a Routine: Incorporate consistent exercise sessions into your weekly timetable. Maintaining consistency is crucial to fully benefit from exercise as a treatment for insulin resistance.

5. Intersperse brief spurts of activity throughout the day to maintain a healthy level of physical activity. During pauses, ascend the stairs, go for a brief stroll, or perform some stretching at your workstation.

It is imperative to seek guidance from a healthcare professional or fitness expert before commencing a new exercise regimen, particularly if you have pre-existing health conditions.

Alterations To One's Lifestyle To Control Insulin Resistance: Beyond Diet And Exercise

Lifestyle modifications are equally as important as insulin resistance recipes and consistent exercise when it comes to the efficient management of insulin resistance. These modifications transcend the tangible elements and incorporate a multitude of facets of everyday existence. The following are essential lifestyle adjustments to contemplate:

1. Sufficient Sleep: Give precedence to sound sleep, as it has a direct influence on insulin sensitivity. Aim for seven to nine hours of restful sleep per night.

2. Stress Management: Insulin resistance may be exacerbated by chronic stress. Integrate stress-relieving practices into your daily regimen, such as yoga, meditation, or deep breathing.

3. Maintaining proper hydration is essential for maintaining overall health and a healthy metabolism. Numerous physiological processes—

including nutrient transportation and refuse elimination—require water.

4. Consistent Monitoring: Maintain a consistent record of your blood sugar levels. This elucidates how your dietary and physical activity decisions influence your insulin sensitivity.

5. Consider Cessation of Smoking: Individuals who smoke should contemplate ceasing. Numerous health problems and insulin resistance are linked to smoking. If necessary, seek assistance from healthcare professionals or support groups.

Bear in mind that lifestyle changes are cumulative in nature, and gradual implementation of minor adjustments can result in substantial advancements over an extended period.

Sample Meal Plans For Individuals Resistant To Insulin:

Establishing well-balanced dietary plans is an essential component in the management of insulin resistance. To promote blood sugar stability, these diets should give precedence to whole, nutrient-dense foods. The following is an example of a daily diet plan tailored to individuals who are undergoing insulin resistance management:

For breakfast,

• Scrambled eggs accompanied by tomatoes and spinach

• Toasted whole grains

• Berries, including strawberries and raspberries

Herbal coffee or black tea

Dish for Lunch:

• Grilled chicken salad comprised of cucumber, cherry tomatoes, and a variety of greenery

Quinoa or brown rice substitutes

• Lemon and olive oil vinaigrette

Hydrocarbons or herbal tea

Snack item:

• Greek yogurt topped with chia seeds

Carrot or apple skewers, sliced

Meal: Dinner

• Salmon baked with seasonings and citrus

• Broccoli and cauliflower steamed

The delightful vegetable

Green tea, a

Snack, if required:

• A small quantity of nuts, such as walnuts or almonds

• Herbal unsweetened tea

It is advisable to modify portion sizes to personal requirements and to seek personalized guidance from a registered dietitian or healthcare professional.

A Health-Conscious Grocery Shopping Guide For Insulin-Friendly Ingredients: How To Navigate The Aisles

Although it can be daunting to navigate the grocery store, having a clear strategy can make selecting ingredients that are welcoming to insulin easier. A guide to making informed decisions while buying is as follows:

1. Fresh Produce: Incorporate an assortment of vibrant vegetables, including verdant greens, bell peppers, asparagus, and tomatoes, into your shopping cart. Choose fruits with a low glycemic index, such as pears, apples, and berries.

2. Lean Proteins: Opt for lean sources of protein such as eggs, skinless poultry, seafood, tofu, and legumes. These sources deliver vital amino acids while avoiding an overabundance of saturated lipids.

3. Opt for whole cereals in your diet, including products made with quinoa, brown rice, oats, and whole wheat. The glycemic index of these cereals is inferior to that of refined grains.

4. To optimize nutritional value, integrate sources of healthy lipids into your diet, including avocados, almonds, seeds, and olive oil. In addition to promoting satiety, these lipids supply vital nutrients.

5. Dairy or Dairy Substitutes: Opt for dairy products that are low in fat or fat-free, or for non-dairy alternatives such as soy milk or almond milk. These alternatives contain calcium and vitamin D without the addition of sugar.

6. Instead of relying excessively on sugar or sodium, augment the flavor of your dishes by utilizing herbs and seasonings. Infusing your dishes with fresh herbs such as basil, cilantro, and mint can increase their vibrancy.

7. It is advisable to restrict one's consumption of refined foods, sugary treats, and sweetened beverages. These may cause sharp increases in blood glucose levels.

8. It is imperative to carefully examine food labels, paying particular attention to the

information provided about added sugars and concealed carbohydrates. Opt for goods that undergo minimal processing and comprise identifiable constituents.

9. Stock up on herbal infusions, water, and other low-calorie beverages to maintain proper hydration. Replace sugary beverages with alternatives that promote adequate hydration.

10. Engage in Preparation: Before visiting the store, generate a shopping list with an emphasis on whole foods, thereby preventing impulsive buying. Strategic planning can assist in maintaining adherence to an insulin-friendly diet.

By implementing these grocery purchasing practices, one can consciously select items that are by their objectives for managing insulin resistance.

As a result, insulin resistance management necessitates a comprehensive strategy encompassing adjustments to one's diet, exercise regimen, and overall way of life. A judicious approach to grocery purchasing, incorporating insulin-resistance recipes, engaging in regular physical activity, and maintaining a balanced meal plan can all contribute to enhanced health and insulin sensitivity. It is highly advisable to seek guidance from healthcare professionals, such as registered dietitians and fitness experts, to customize these strategies to suit your specific requirements and situation.

CHAPTER FOUR

Insulin Resistance Recipes: Balanced Nutrition For The Body

Insulin resistance, characterized by diminished cellular responsiveness to insulin's effects, can have profound implications for an individual's overall well-being.

Diet is a critical factor in the management of insulin resistance; therefore, the development of recipes for individuals with insulin resistance requires the use of culinary methods that promote blood sugar regulation and the selection of nutrient-dense ingredients. In this article, we investigate recipes for individuals with insulin resistance, including delectable dishes, culinary techniques, and ingredients that support metabolic health.

Components Rich In Nutrients

1. Include in your preparations an assortment of verdant greens, such as Swiss chard, kale, and spinach. These leafy greens are an excellent source of vitamins, minerals, and fiber, all of

which promote general health and aid in blood sugar regulation.

2. Lean protein sources, including chicken, turkey, fish, and tofu, should be prioritized. Protein promotes satiety and aids in blood sugar regulation, thereby decreasing the likelihood of gorging.

3. Incorporate nutritious lipids into your diet, such as avocados, almonds, and olive oil. These lipids facilitate the absorption of fat-soluble vitamins and promote satiety.

4. Opt for whole grains over refined cereals, such as quinoa, brown rice, and oats. The presence of fiber in whole cereals aids in the regulation of blood sugar levels by impeding the absorption of sugar.

5. A variety of vibrant vegetables should be incorporated into the diet to guarantee a comprehensive assortment of nutrients. Carrots, bell peppers, and tomatoes contribute not only

flavor but also vital nutrients in the form of vitamins and antioxidants.

6. Berries are low in sugar and rich in antioxidants; blueberries, strawberries, and raspberries are examples. They are outstanding in salads, smoothies, and as a nutritious dessert alternative.

7. Legumes: Chickpeas, lentils, and beans are all superb sources of plant-based protein and fiber. They promote satiety and aid in blood sugar regulation.

8. In addition to imparting a pleasant taste, cinnamon has been associated with enhanced insulin sensitivity. Utilize cinnamon in savory dishes or sprinkle it on yogurt or oatmeal.

Techniques Of Preparation For Insulin Resistance

1. Vegetables are preserved in their nutritional value and their natural flavors are enhanced through the process of steaming. It is a fast and

effortless method for preparing nutrient-dense side vegetables.

2. By grilling lean proteins such as fish and chicken, a charred flavor can be achieved without the addition of excessive lipids. Be cautious, however, when marinating in sauces loaded with sugar.

3. The natural carbohydrates in vegetables are caramelized during roasting, which enhances their flavor. Herbs and olive oil should be used to toss them for a nutritious and flavorful side dish.

4. Stir-frying should be performed with minimal oil to maintain the crispiness of vegetables. For a well-balanced meal, incorporate a variety of vibrant vegetables and lean proteins.

5. By baking lean proteins and whole cereals, one can create a nutritious and simple-to-prepare dish. Herb-seasoned chicken breasts or baked sweet potatoes can be both delectable and low in glucose.

6. When cooking, utilize heart-healthy lipids such as olive oil to brown proteins or vegetables. Incorporate herbs, garlic, or ginger for flavoring purposes, avoiding the use of excessive amounts of salt or sugar.

7. Slow cooking permits the fusion of flavors and frequently reduces the amount of added lipids and sugars in a dish. Incorporate an assortment of lean proteins, legumes, and vegetables into substantial stews and soups.

Facts And Common Myths Regarding Insulin Resistance

1. Fallacy No. 1: All Carbohydrates Are Adverse to Insulin Resistance

• It is a fact that carbohydrates vary in quality. Prioritize the consumption of fruits, vegetables, and whole grains, as they contain fiber and vital nutrients. It is essential to avoid refined carbohydrates to control insulin resistance.

2. Insulin resistance specifically affects those who are overweight.

• In contrast to obesity, which is a risk factor, individuals of any weight can develop insulin resistance. Its development is influenced by genetic factors, sedentary occupations, and poor dietary decisions.

3. Contrary to popular belief, insulin resistance is reversible.

Insulin resistance can be ameliorated through the maintenance of a healthy weight, incorporation of a well-balanced diet, and consistent engagement in physical activity. Maintenance of a healthful diet can have a beneficial effect on insulin sensitivity.

4. Insulin resistance is solely caused by sugar consumption.

• It is true that although an inordinate consumption of sugar does contribute to insulin resistance, it is not the only determinant. Lack of physical activity, a diet high in saturated lipids, and genetic predisposition are additional influential factors.

5. Myth: Young people are not affected by insulin resistance.

Insulin resistance can manifest at any stage of life. Younger individuals are progressively more vulnerable due to the acceleration of sedentary lifestyles and the adoption of unhealthy dietary practices.

6. Insulin resistance causes diabetes invariably.

• It is not true that all individuals with insulin resistance progress to type 2 diabetes, even though it is a precursor to the condition. Lifestyle modifications have the potential to impede or postpone the progression of the condition.

FAQs: Frequently Asked Questions

1. Does insulin resistance preclude the consumption of desserts?

• A: You may, but choose healthful alternatives instead. Replace refined flours with natural sweeteners such as stevia or monk fruit, and experiment with recipes that call for almond flour or cereals.

2. How critical is portion control in the management of type 2 diabetes?

Portion control is an essential factor. Throughout the day, consuming fewer, more balanced meals helps regulate blood sugar levels. Avoid eating frequently and in significant quantities, as this can cause blood sugar surges.

3. Are there any particular nutrients that have the potential to enhance insulin sensitivity?

• In fact, there is evidence to suggest that consuming oily salmon (which are abundant in omega-3 fatty acids), leafy vegetables, and foods high in magnesium (such as nuts and seeds) may enhance insulin sensitivity.

4. Exercise as a management strategy for insulin resistance?

Consistent physical activity is, in fact, vital. Resistance training and aerobic exercise are both effective in enhancing insulin sensitivity and regulating blood sugar levels.

5. Can a low-carbohydrate diet be utilized to control insulin resistance?

Although low-carb diets may be effective for some individuals, it is crucial to prioritize the quality of carbohydrates consumed. For balanced and sustainable nutrition, select complex carbohydrates and watch your overall caloric intake.

In summary, the process of developing recipes for individuals with insulin resistance entails the careful selection of ingredients that are rich in nutrients, the application of methodical culinary approaches, and the debunking of prevalent misconceptions. Through the adoption of a well-rounded and nutritious dietary philosophy, individuals can enhance their capacity to regulate insulin resistance and foster holistic health.

Conclusion

In summary, implementing insulin resistance recipes represents an empowering and proactive strategy for addressing and alleviating the consequences of insulin resistance.

These recipes give precedence to whole foods that are rich in nutrients and aid in the regulation of blood sugar, reduction of inflammation, and promotion of general health.

These recipes promote enhanced insulin sensitivity through the utilization of a well-balanced combination of lean proteins, healthy lipids, and complex carbohydrates.

The consumption of foods abundant in fiber facilitates the deceleration of glucose assimilation, thereby averting abrupt increases in blood sugar levels. Additionally, the inclusion of components abundant in antioxidants can mitigate oxidative stress, a contributory element to insulin resistance.

Diabetes-friendly recipes are sustainable for long-term adherence due to their adaptability and palatability. In addition to promoting metabolic health, incorporating a wide variety of fruits, vegetables, whole cereals, and lean proteins into one's diet enhances the palatability and taste of food. Furthermore, these recipes advocate for a reduction in the consumption of processed and refined foods, thereby encouraging the adoption of a more nutritious and health-conscious dietary regimen.

In essence, the endeavor to counteract insulin resistance via gastronomic selections encompasses not only the maintenance of a medical condition but also the cultivation of a comprehensive and pleasurable dietary philosophy. By incorporating methods for managing insulin resistance into their daily routines, people can proactively enhance their overall health and wellness.

THE END